Himalayan Salt

Himalayan Salt

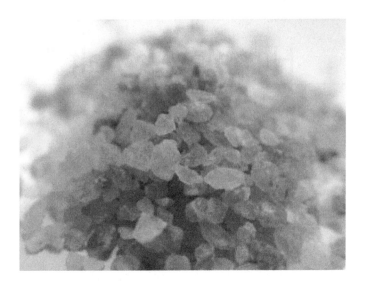

A Complete User's Guide

Including types of Himalayan salt, benefits,
cooking tips, recipes, health information and more.

Author: Aysel Us

ISBN 978-0-9925420-1-6

Printed by Lightning Source, Victoria

Disclaimer

Although the author and publisher have made every effort to ensure that the information in this book was correct at press time, the author and publisher do not assume and hereby disclaim any liability to any party for any loss, injury, damage or disruption caused by errors or omissions, whether such errors or omissions result from negligence, accident, non-functional websites, or any other cause. Any advice or strategy contained herein may not be suitable for every individual.

Foreword

When you think of salt you probably imagine those tiny white crystals you find in the salt shaker on your kitchen table. That form of salt is highly refined and, in all honesty, bad for you. Real salt like Himalayan Salt is loaded with natural minerals that provide significant health advantages for your body. If you are curious about the dangers of table salt and how Himalayan Salt can benefit you, this book is the perfect place to start.

Written in a clear and easy-to-read fashion, this book on Himalayan Salt provides you with background knowledge on what Himalayan Salt is and where it comes from. You will also learn the basics about what this type of salt is used for and how it can benefit your body. Additionally, you will receive a collection of recipes for making food and homemade bath-and-body products with all-natural Himalayan Salt. If you are ready to discover the secret of Himalayan Salt, keep reading!

Acknowledgements

I would like to extend my sincerest thanks to my family for their endless support as I pursue my writing endeavors. And thanks to all those who contributed their favorite recipes for inclusion in this book.

Table of Contents

Chapter One: Introduction

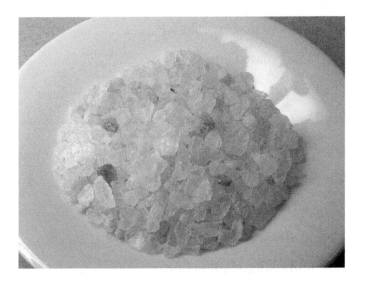

In the health and fitness world, there is always a new trend or fad hitting the market. Whether it is a new cleanse or some kind of super food, people are eager to jump on board, regardless whether the trend is supported by scientific evidence or not. If you have experienced this phenomenon or have heard about it yourself, you may be skeptical about the claimed benefits of Himalayan Salt. After all, salt is bad for you – isn't it?

The truth of the matter is that many people's perception of salt is entirely wrong. Not only is salt (in the right form) good for you, but it is actually necessary for your body to function properly. This isn't to say that you should pour table salt onto every meal you eat. In fact, table salt is part of the problem that leads people to believe that all salt is bad. Himalayan Salt, on the other hand, is completely pure – free from toxins and made up of 84 minerals that are naturally found in the human body.

In this book you will learn all about Himalayan Salt including the basics of what it is and where it comes from to specifics about its health benefits. This wonderful mineral has the power to balance fluid levels in the body, reduce the signs of aging, increase bone strength and to promote healthy sleep patterns. Within the pages of this book you will learn about all of these health benefits and more – you will also read about the uses for Himalayan Salt in cooking and receive a collection of delicious recipes to try for yourself at home.

Useful Terms to Know

Ayurvedic Medicine – also known simply as Ayurveda, a type of traditional Hindu medicine native to the Indian subcontinent

Composition – the chemical make-up of a substance; the relative amounts of various elements that constitute a single substance

Halite – also known as rock salt; the natural mineral form of sodium chloride; typically colorless but may be black, blue, pink, red, or yellow depending on the impurities

Himalayas – a large mountain range in Asia that separates the Indian subcontinent from the Tibetan plateau; runs for 1,500 miles (2,400 km) between Nanga Parbat in the west and Namcha Barwa in the east

Mineral – a naturally occurring substance that is solid at room temperature; has an ordered atomic structure and a specific chemical formula

Rock Salt – the natural form of salt as a crystalline mineral, also known as halite

Salt Slab – a solid piece of salt often used for cooking by heating it slowly over low heat

Salt Lamp – a large hollowed-out piece of salt outfitted with a low-wattage bulb that heats the salt to release negative ions into the air

Salt Range – a hill system in the Punjab province of Pakistan where large deposits of natural salt can be found

Sodium Chloride – an ionic compound produced from equal portions of sodium and chlorine; common name is salt or halite

Chapter Two: Understanding Himalayan Salt

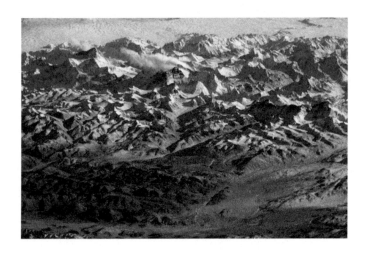

As you can probably guess from the name, Himalayan Salt comes from the Himalayas (pictured above), a mountain range that spans more than 1,500 miles (2,400 km) in Asia. However, there is so much more to learn about this amazing mineral. In this chapter you will learn the basics about sea salt, including Himalayan Salt, as well as information about its mineral composition, how it is collected and what it can be used for. By the time you finish this chapter you will have a good basic understanding of Himalayan Salt.

1.) What is Sea Salt?

You are probably familiar with salt, the white substance that you use to flavor food, but you may not be as familiar with sea salt. Sea salt is produced through the evaporation of saltwater (seawater) and it can be used for a variety of purposes, not just for cooking. Sea salt has been produced for centuries – in fact, the earliest mentions of it come from the Vinaya Pitaka, a Buddhist scripture that was written in the mid-5th century BC.

Other Names for Salt

Sodium chloride

Bay Salt (sea salt)

Solar Salt (sea salt)

Halite (Himalayan Salt)

Rock Salt (Himalayan Salt)

Himalayan Crystal Salt

For thousands of years, sea salt has played an important role in human history. During the times of ancient Egypt, it was used in religious ceremonies and for trade with the Phoenicians. In fact, salt was so valuable that it was utilized as a form of currency in many areas. At one time, salt was traded ounce-per-ounce with gold – if that were still the case today, you would be paying $300 (£195) or more per ounce of salt. The modern word "salary" comes from the word "salt" which is just one more testament to the importance of this mineral throughout human history.

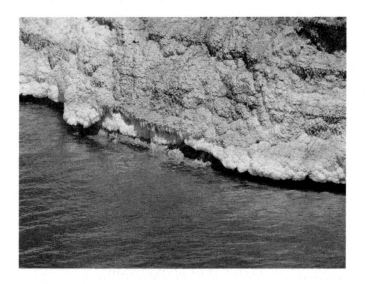

Sea salt exists in many forms but one of the most popular types is Himalayan Salt, also known as halite. This type of salt comes largely from Pakistan and its origins lie in the Primal Sea, an underground sea located deep within the Himalayan Mountains that was formed about 250 million years ago. What was once a sea dried up over thousands of years, leaving large deposits of pure, crystal-like salt that is now known as Himalayan Salt. The salt is chipped out of large salt formations and used to create a variety of products like salt lamps, bath salts, and even salts for cooking and natural remedies.

a.) Mineral Composition

As you are probably already aware, different minerals have different chemical compositions – all minerals are made up of various ions. What makes Himalayan Salt so interesting is that it contains 84 different naturally-occurring minerals, many of which are essential for maintaining optimal health. Himalayan Salt contains about 98% sodium chloride, 0.07% magnesium, 0.05% sulfate and about 0.0006% iron.

A full list of the minerals found in Himalayan Salt is as follows:

Hydrogen	Fluoride	Chloride
Lithium	Sodium	Potassium
Beryllium	Magnesium	Calcium
Boron	Aluminum	Scandium
Carbon	Silicon	Titanium
Nitrogen	Phosphorus	Vanadium
Oxygen	Sulfur	Chromium

Manganese	Palladium	Holmium
Iron	Silver	Erbium
Cobalt	Cadmium	Thulium
Nickel	Indium	Ytterbium
Copper	Tin	Lutetium
Zinc	Antimony	Hafnium
Gallium	Tellurium	Tantalum
Germanium	Iodine	Wolfram
Arsenic	Cesium	Rhenium
Selenium	Barium	Osmium
Bromine	Lanthanum	Iridium
Rubidium	Cerium	Platinum
Strontium	Praseodymium	Gold
Ytterbium	Neodymium	Mercury
Zirconium	Promethium	Thallium
Niobium	Samarium	Lead
Molybdenum	Europium	Bismuth
Technetium	Gadolinium	Polonium
Ruthenium	Terbium	Astatine
Rhodium	Dysprosium	Francium

Radium	Protactinium	Plutonium
Actinium	Uranium	
Thorium	Neptunium	

<u>To give you a frame of reference for comparing Himalayan Salt to other salts, consider this:</u>

- Table salt contains about 97.5% sodium chloride and 2.5% other chemicals including iodine and absorbents.

- Pink rose salt contains about 95.5% sodium chloride, 0.02% magnesium, 0.64% potassium, and 0.07% calcium.

- Black lava salt contains 0.34% magnesium, 0.20% potassium, and 35.94% sodium.

2.) Where Does it Come From?

The Khewra Salt Mine is the largest source of Himalayan Salt in the world and the second largest salt mine in general. This mine is located in Khewra which belongs to the Jhelum District in Pakistan. The mine is located about 125 miles (200 km) from Lahore and Islamabad within a mineral-rich mountain range that extends for more than 125 miles (200 km) throughout Pakistan from the Jehlum River to where it joins with the Indus River. The mine itself is the largest and oldest mine in Pakistan and a major tourist attraction, hosting as many as 250,000 visitors per year.

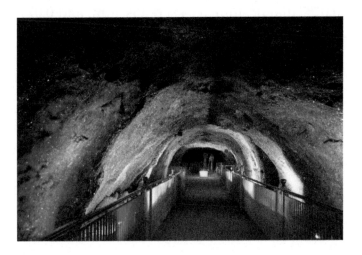

The Khewra Salt Mine was discovered by Alexander the Great's troops as early as 320 BC but it didn't start trading until the age of the Mughal Empire during the 16th century. The salt range in which the mine is located was formed over 800 million years ago by the evaporation of a shallow underground sea. The geological movement that followed led to the formation of a salt range that extends more than 185 miles (300 km). The credit for the discovery of the salt range does not go to Alexander the Great himself, nor to his troops – it goes to his horses that were found licking the stones in the area.

During the age of the Mughal Empire in the 16th century, salt from the range was traded in markets all over the continent, as far away as Central Asia. When the Mughal Empire fell, the mine was taken over by the Sikhs. The mine was divided into two sections – Hari Singh Nalwa, the Sikh Commander-in-Chief, was given control of the Warcha mine; while Gulab Singh, the Raja of Jammu, was given control of the Khewru mine. Throughout the time the mine was controlled by the Sikhs, its salt was used for both food and as a source of revenue through trade.

By the last 1800s, the British Empire had taken control of the mine and developed it further. The narrow, irregular tunnels within the mine were found to be inefficient and the quality of the water supply within the mine was very poor. Over the decades that followed, the British levelled the road leading to the mine to make access easier, built warehouses for storage, improved the water supply and introduced improved means for the excavation of salt from the mine.

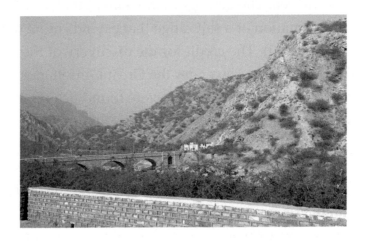

Given the size of the Khewra Salt Mine, it is difficult to calculate how much salt the salt range actually contains. Estimates of the reserves in the mine, however, come in at a minimum of 82 million tons and a maximum around 600 million tons. The mine is currently controlled by the Pakistan Mineral Development Corporation and produces about 350,000 tons of salt per year. This number is greatly increased from the output during British rule which was only around 28,000 to 30,000 tons per year. The current rate of production for the mine amounts to nearly half of the total rock salt production in Pakistan and it is estimated that the mine will last another 350 years at this rate.

3.) What are its Uses?

Himalayan Salt is an incredibly versatile mineral that can be used for a variety of purposes. The most common uses of this mineral are for culinary or medicinal purposes. Himalayan Salt, however, can also be used for food preservation and for the production of salt lamps and salt slabs. You will read more about all of these uses in the following pages of this section.

a.) Cooking

Himalayan Salt for cooking comes in a wide variety of forms including coarse grain, small grain, fine grain, powder, and more. Because there are so many different types of Himalayan Salt, you can choose the one that is ideal for your cooking purposes. <u>Below you will find a list of the types of salt available and what type of dishes they are best suited for</u>:

Coarse Grain – Extra course and coarse grain rock salt like Himalayan Salt is ideal for use in salt mills and grinders if you want freshly ground salt to flavor a dish. This type of salt is also great for roasting, grilling and curing meats.

Medium Grain – A medium-grain Himalayan Salt can also be used in smaller grinders as well as for roasting meat. This type of salt is also recommended for making brine and spice rubs before cooking meat.

Small/Fine Grain – In addition to being good for spice rubs and roasting, small or fine-grain Himalayan Salt can be sprinkled directly on food for seasoning before or after cooking. Fine-grain salt can also be used for rimming the glass when making specialty cocktails.

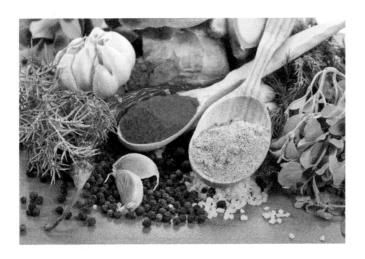

Powder (Extra-Fine) – Powdered Himalayan Salt is very fine and works very well for most cooking applications including grilling, roasting and seasoning. This grain of salt is the best for salt shakers.

Another way to use Himalayan Salt for cooking is to cook foods directly on salt slabs. You will read more about this later in this section.

b.) Health

You already know that Himalayan Salt contains 84 different minerals that are essential for optimal health in the human body. Incorporating Himalayan Salt in your cooking recipes can have a variety of health benefits including the following:

- Improves brain function and mental clarity
- Rids the body of toxic wastes that speed aging
- Eases cramps and digestive problems
- Regulates fluid levels in the body, promotes balance
- Purifies and detoxifies the blood
- Replenishes levels of vital electrolytes
- Supports healthy vascular and respiratory function
- Naturally promotes healthy sleep patterns
- Increases libido supports sexual vitality
- Helps the body absorb nutrients more efficiently

In addition to providing these health benefits for your body when consumed, Himalayan Salt can also be used in a variety of bath and spa products. Taking a bath with Himalayan Salt can be incredibly beneficial for your skin as it helps to balance your body's energy flow. To use Himalayan Salt correctly in a bath you should use hot water (around 97°F/37°C) and a concentration of about 1.28 ounces of salt per gallon of water. Soak for at least 20 to 30 minutes and do not rinse off afterward – just towel dry. To gain the maximum benefit, rest for 30 minutes after your bath before you continue your daily activities.

c.) Salt Lamps

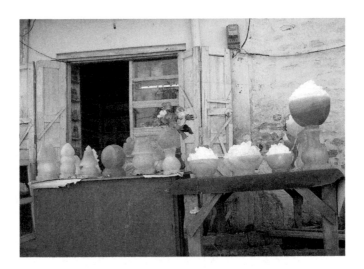

Another unique way to experience the benefits of Himalayan Salt is through a salt lamp. A salt lamp simply consists of slab of Himalayan Salt with a low-wattage light bulb inserted in the center. When the lamp is turned on, the bulb gently heats the salt which causes it to emit negative ions in the air. Negative ions provide a number of benefits including the removal of dust, cigarette smoke, pollen and bacteria from the air – it also offsets the positive ions that are emitted by your TV, computer monitor and other electronic devices.

To get the most out of your salt lamp, it is important that you choose the proper placement. Ideally, you should place several lamps throughout your home in the areas you and your family frequent – the living room, office, bedroom, etc. In addition to providing you with the benefits of negative ions, having salt lamps spaced throughout your home will also add to the beauty and serenity of your home.

d.) Food Preservation

In addition to using Himalayan Salt to flavor food, it can also be used to preserve it. The method used to preserve food with Himalayan Salt is called curing and it is best used on meat, fish and vegetables. This food preservation method is an ancient one, dating back to before the invention of modern preservation methods like refrigeration and even ice boxes. In fact, scientific evidence has been found to support the use of Himalayan Salt for food preservation since before the last ice age which occurred over 12,000 years ago. Properly cured foods can last for weeks or months without refrigeration.

e.) Salt Slabs

As was mentioned earlier, salt slabs are another way to cook with Himalayan Salt. A salt slab is simply a cut block of Himalayan Salt that can be placed directly on the burner of your stove. To use a salt slab for cooking, follow the instructions below:

1. Place the salt slab directly on the burner of a gas range or use a metal ring (like a tart pan with a removable bottom) to elevate the slab just above the burner.
2. Turn the burner on to the lowest heat setting possible and let it heat for 15 minutes until the slab reaches about 200°F/93°C.
3. Increase the heat slightly every 10 minutes, moving from low to medium and from medium to high.
4. Once the block reaches 500°F/260°C you can add your meat directly to the block.

Tip: For the best results, your meat should be cut into thin strips no more than a few inches long. Flip the meat halfway through and cook to the desired level.

Chapter Three: Types of Himalayan Salt

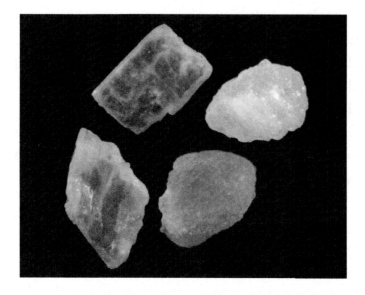

Now that you understand the basics about sea salt, and Himalayan Salt in particular, you may be curious about some of the specifics regarding this amazing mineral. There are several different types of Himalayan Salt including pink and black Himalayan Salt which you will learn more about in this chapter. Also in this chapter you will learn what differentiates Himalayan Salt from other types of sea salt like Celtic sea salt.

1.) Pink Himalayan Salt

Pink Himalayan Salt is a type of rock salt, or halite, which formed as a crystalline mineral in large deposits in the Himalayas. You have already read a great deal about pink Himalayan Salt because it is the most common type of Himalayan salt. This type of salt can be used to flavor foods, in food preservation, for natural remedies and for various other purposes such as salt lamps and salt slabs that are used for cooking.

This type of Himalayan Salt is often regarded as the purest form of salt due to its high mineral content. The color of pink Himalayan Salt ranges from deep red to light pink depending on the mineral concentration. The pink color of this salt is specifically due to the presence of trace elements including iron. Some of the other key elements found in pink Himalayan Salt include calcium, magnesium, copper and potassium. All of these minerals work together to provide a number of unique and significant health benefits.

Some of the health benefits specific to pink Himalayan Salt include:

- Balancing the pH of the body
- Normalizing low or high blood pressure
- Increasing circulation of the blood

- Eliminating toxins from the blood and body
- Improving absorption of nutrients
- Relieving arthritis pain
- Balancing electrolytes in the body.

You will read more about the specific benefits and uses of pink Himalayan Salt later in this book.

2.) Black Himalayan Salt (Kala Namak)

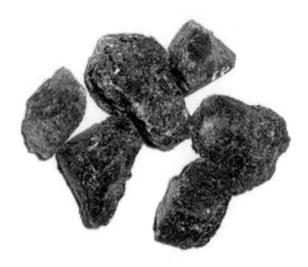

This type of Himalayan Salt is known by many different names including the following:

- Kala Namak
- Sulemani Namak
- Black Salt
- Kala Loon
- Black Indian Salt

Essentially, black Himalayan Salt is a type of rock salt that is derived from natural halite formations throughout the

Himalayan salt ranges in Pakistan, Nepal, India and Bangladesh. It can also be harvested from the North Indian salt lakes in the Sambhar, Didwana and Mustang areas of Nepal. This type of salt is commonly used as a condiment throughout South Asia, known for its dark color and pungent smell. The smell is due to the salt's high concentration of sulfur.

Black Himalayan Salt was traditionally transformed from its raw form into a new form for commercial purposes using a reductive chemical process that involved firing the salt for 24 hours. During firing, the salt was sealed in a ceramic jar along with charcoal and various seeds. After firing, the salt was then cooled, stored and aged. This preparation method is partially what gives the salt its black color. In its raw form, however, this type of Himalayan Salt still has a brownish pink hue due to the presence of impurities and various trace minerals.

a.) Chemical Composition

Black Himalayan Salt, like pink Himalayan Salt, is largely comprised of sodium chloride. The difference between the two lies in the trace minerals and impurities. Black Himalayan Salt contains trace amounts of sodium sulphate, sodium bisulfate, sodium bisulfite, sodium sulphide, iron sulfide and hydrogen sulfide. The sodium chloride concentration is what gives black Himalayan Salt its salty taste while the iron sulphide provides the dark brownish red hue. All of the sulphur compounds in the salt give it a sulfuric smell and a savory taste.

Note: Hydrogen sulphide is a toxic compound in high concentrations but the concentration of this compound in black Himalayan Salt is not high enough to be dangerous for human consumption.

b.) Uses for Black Himalayan Salt

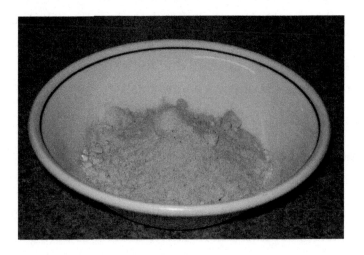

As you can see from the picture above, black Himalayan Salt still has a largely pink color when it is ground into powder. It is only the raw form of the salt that maintains its dark brownish red color. This type of salt can be used in all of its forms for a variety of culinary purposes, particularly in South Asian cuisine. In India, Pakistan and Bangladesh, black Himalayan Salt is used as a condiment to flavor chutneys, salads, chaats, raitas and other dishes. In India, it is a key element in Chaat masala, a traditional spice blend.

In addition to its culinary uses, black Himalayan Salt also serves a variety of purposes in Ayurvedic medicine. It has been used as a laxative and digestive aid as well as to relieve gas and heartburn. When combined with other plant ingredients, this salt makes a good toothpaste and it has also been used to treat hysteria. In Jammu, a district in India, it has long been used to cure goiters.

3.) Himalayan Salt vs. Celtic Sea Salt

Celtic sea salt is also known as *sel gris* or "gray salt" in French. This type of salt is coarse and granular with a higher moisture percentage than many salts – it contains about 13% residual moisture compared to the 0.026% residual moisture found in Himalayan Salt. In addition to its different mineral composition, the harvesting methods for Celtic sea salt differ from those used for Himalayan Salt. It is typically gathered by evaporating seawater and collecting the salt in a salt pan.

Like Himalayan Salt, Celtic sea salt can be used for a variety of different purposes. This salt has a fairly coarse grain but it can be used for both cooking and finishing. It is important to keep in mind, however, that the density of Celtic sea salt is much greater than traditional table salt so you do not need to use as much of it. Celtic sea salt also has a lot of residual moisture in it, so it will not suck the moisture out of food.

a.) Mineral Composition

In comparison to Himalayan Salt, Celtic sea salt only contains about 34 trace minerals, though refined Celtic sea salt may have additional minerals added. Celtic sea salt

contains about 84% sodium chloride in comparison to
Himalayan Salt's 98% concentration. This is due to the fact
that Celtic Sea Salt contains a higher amount of natural
brine (seawater) which lowers the concentration of sodium
chloride. Though the number of trace minerals found in
Celtic Sea Salt is lower than for Himalayan Salt, the total
concentration of these minerals is higher (between 15 and
23% versus 2 to 4%).

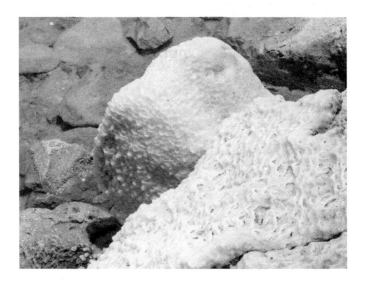

b.) Celtic vs. Himalayan Salt

Now that you know the basics about Celtic sea salt you may
be wondering what makes Himalayan Salt better. After all,
Celtic sea salt has a higher concentration of trace minerals,

though the number of minerals present may be a little lower. The main difference between the two is purity – Himalayan Salt is over 99% pure whereas Celtic sea salt typically contains impurities and can easily be contaminated during harvesting. Himalayan Salt is completely unrefined and requires no refinement or processing to be edible.

Throughout this book you will learn more details about why Himalayan Salt is good for you and what kind of benefits it can provide for your body.

Chapter Four: The Role of Salt in the Body

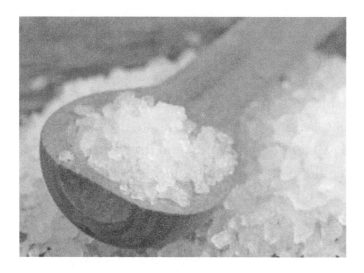

As you already know, your body is made up of complex systems that work together in clearly defined ways. Everything you put into your body (and those things that you deprive it of) has an impact on your body's function and on your health. In this chapter you will learn about the role that salt plays in your body and how some of the specific minerals it contains can impact your health. More specifically, you will learn why Himalayan Salt is the best salt to use in order to preserve your health.

1.) Balancing Body Fluids

When you think of hydration, you probably think of water. What you may not realize, however, is that salt also plays a key role in keeping your body hydrated. More specifically, salt plays an important role in keeping the fluid balance both inside and outside of your cells. So, while drinking water is essential for good hydration, if you do not consume natural salt as well you could end up with a fluid imbalance which could lead to health problems including hypernatremia.

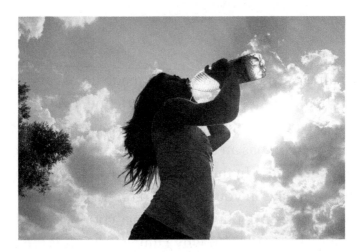

The concept of fluid balance in the body relates to the ratio of water intake to water loss – in order to achieve balance, the amount of fluid you take in each day should be equivalent to the amount of fluid your body excretes. The average adult male requires about 3.7 liters of water per day while an adult female needs about 2.7 liters per day. Food consumption contributes to between 0.5 and 1 liter of water per day and the rest comes from drinking water.

The major aspect of fluid excretion, or loss, during the day is urination – the average person urinates about 4 times per day. Other methods of fluid output include perspiration (sweating), respiration and, in females, vaginal secretions. The rate of fluid output is regulated by certain hormones in the body – these hormones include ADH (antidiuretic hormone) and aldosterone.

In terms of fluid balance, salt comes into play in conjunction with electrolyte levels. Sodium is the main type of electrolyte found in extracellular fluid, and it plays a major role in maintaining both blood pressure and fluid balance in the cells. As you sweat, your body loses electrolytes which can impact your overall fluid balance. Thus, you need to consume salt in order to replenish your electrolyte stores and to restore fluid balance in the body.

2.) Salt and Magnesium

Magnesium is one of many essential minerals found in Himalayan Salt and it provides very significant benefits for the body. One of the main constituents of living matter, magnesium helps to regulate the activity of more than 300 different enzymes in the human body. Magnesium deficiency has been linked to a number of health problems including the following:

- High blood pressure
- Decalcification of bones
- Hyperactivity
- Rapid weight loss
- Heart disease
- Dizziness
- Irritability and mood swings

So what exactly does magnesium do in the body? Magnesium is a type of mineral that has a charge of plus 2 when broken down in the body – that makes it a divalent cation. The main role of this cation is to regulate enzyme function – it is a cofactor that allows chemical reactions to take place in the body without damaging the surrounding tissues with heat or acid production. If magnesium were not present to regulate these reactions, they could wreak havoc on the body and cause very real damage.

Magnesium is also an important element in the production of energy in the body. ATP, adenosine triphosphate, is the type of energy your cells use to reproduce, to synthesize proteins and to transport substances. Without magnesium, units of ATP could not be efficiently metabolized and used for energy. This is why magnesium deficiency often leads to the calcification of bones and tissues as well as muscular symptoms like cramps and spasms.

In reference to the previous section, magnesium also plays a role in fluid balance within the body. In order to achieve proper fluid balance, the concentration of magnesium must be high inside the cell and low outside the cell. Magnesium also plays a role in balancing sodium-potassium levels, as you will read in the next section. For all of the reasons discussed, having adequate levels of magnesium in your body is very important – particularly in conjunction with sodium and potassium levels. Himalayan Salt contains magnesium at a concentration of 0.16 g/kg.

3.) Potassium in Salt

Potassium is one of several macrominerals found in abundance in Himalayan Salt and it is very important for your health. More specifically, the balance of sodium and potassium in your body is essential for cardiovascular health. If your diet is too high in sodium without complementary amounts of potassium, you could experience a number of health problems including high blood pressure and various forms of heart disease.

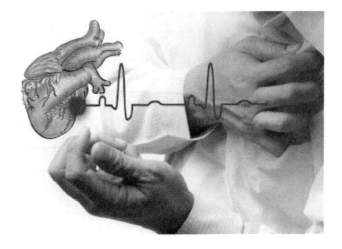

The mineral potassium serves as an electrolyte in the human body along with sodium and chloride. An electrolyte is an atom that carries an electrical charge and transmits that electricity to create muscle contractions and to facilitate nerve communication in the brain. While chloride has a negative ionic charge, both sodium and potassium are positively charged. The difference is that sodium is more highly concentrated outside the cells (extracellular) while potassium is highly concentrated in the cells (intracellular). When the concentrations of these ions are balanced inside and outside the cells, it facilitates the smooth flow of electrical currents and fluid.

As you already know, fluid balance is essential for good health. When your sodium and potassium levels become imbalanced, your body may start to retain water in an effort to maintain fluid levels. This, in turn, increases your blood volume which leads to an increase in blood pressure. The latter, then, affects the pumping of your heart. Over time, excess sodium intake without adequate potassium intake to balance it can lead to chronic high blood pressure which will increase your risk of heart disease and stroke. Using a natural salt like Himalayan Salt that contains potassium, rather than table salt which has had its potassium content removed, can help to maintain the balance of sodium and potassium in the human body.

4.) The Importance of Iodine

Iodine is a mineral that tends to collect in oceans and brine pools – this explains its presence in Himalayan Salt. This element is incredibly important for human health and deficiency can lead to a number of severe problems including the following:

- Hypothyroidism
- Goiters
- Mental deficiency
- Stunted growth
- Slowed metabolism
- Certain forms of cancer

The most important function of iodine is to regulate the production of hormones in the thyroid gland. These hormones are responsible for controlling your metabolism as well as the growth and development of your bones, brain and tissues. The hormones produced by your thyroid are essential for controlling the production and utilization of energy in nearly every cell of your body, so you can see why it is so important.

Iodine deficiency is a very serious problem, and one that is on the rise particularly in the United States. Discoveries about iodine deficiency are what prompted the addition of iodine to table salt during the 1920s. Unfortunately, the type of iodine added to table salt (a synthetic form called iodide) is not as easily utilized by the body. Himalayan Salt, however, contains natural iodine which the body can use easily in the production and transport of hormones.

You may find it interesting to learn how iodine deficiency affects certain tissues in your body. <u>Below you will find a chart relating the symptoms of iodine deficiency in certain types of tissue</u>:

Tissue	Symptoms of Deficiency
Brain	Reduced cognitive function and alertness, lowered IQ
Muscles	Pain, fibrosis, fibromyalgia, scar tissue, formation of nodules
Skin	Dry skin, lack of sweating
Salivary Glands	Dry mouth, inability to produce saliva

To prevent iodine deficiency, you should take the time to learn how much iodine your body needs. The human body is capable of holding up to 1,500 mg of iodine at any given time – the thyroid itself can hold up to 50 mg. Up to 20% of the iodine in your body is contained in your skin while 32% is stored in your muscles. According to the USDA, adult men and women have a recommended daily allowance for iodine around 150 mcg. This number increases to 220 mcg for pregnant women and to 290 for women who are lactating/breastfeeding. Himalayan Salt contains iodine at a concentration of around 0.1g/kg.

a.) Iodine and Selenium

In the human body, the minerals iodine and selenium are closely linked. In fact, selenium is a necessary cofactor for a certain type of enzymes called iodothyronine deiodinases – the enzymes responsible for the activation/deactivation of thyroid hormones. Given the link between these two minerals, it makes sense that selenium deficiency can exacerbate or mimic the symptoms of iodine deficiency. Luckily, Himalayan Salt contains both of these minerals – an iodine concentration of 0.1 g/kg and a selenium concentration of 0.05 ppm.

Chapter Five: Himalayan Salt for Health

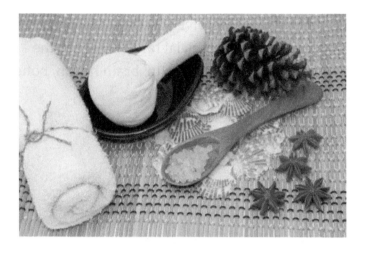

After reading the previous chapter, you already have a good idea what role Himalayan Salt can play in your body. You should not be surprised, then, to learn of the many benefits this mineral has for your health. <u>Some of the many benefits that Himalayan Salt can provide include:</u>

- Balancing blood sugar levels in the body
- Supporting nerve cell communication and information processing in the brain
- Helps to prevent muscle cramps during exercise
- Contributes to bone strength, prevents osteoporosis
- Vital for healthy sleep regulation
- May help to clear up congestion and other minor ailments

- Helps the body absorb nutrients in the intestinal tract

In this chapter you will receive specific information about how Himalayan Salt is beneficial for the body in the following areas: aging, heart health, brain health, bone health and sleep.

1.) Himalayan Salt for Aging

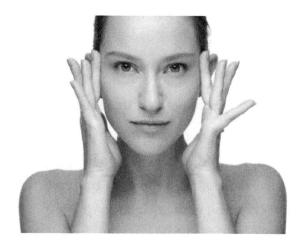

You may already know that the food you eat has a significant impact on your body and, more specifically, on your skin. If you eat an unhealthy diet loaded with saturated fats and deficient in nutrients, your skin is going to show it by looking oily – you may also experience frequent breakouts and you could even develop early wrinkles. Though there are many "miracle products" on the market to reverse the signs of aging, the solution may actually be simpler than you think – Himalayan Salt.

Himalayan Salt can cleanse and detoxify the skin, helping to draw out toxic substances which will leave your skin clear and smooth. The natural minerals in Himalayan Salt can also be beneficial in treating a number of skin conditions including psoriasis, acne and general dry skin – it may also be effective in treating insect bites and blisters. The best way to gain these benefits from Himalayan Salt is to soak in a salt bath.

a.) Tips for Using Himalayan Bath Salts

Himalayan bath salts come in a variety of forms, so the amount you use may vary depending on the product. Some bath salts are very fine while others may be coarse ground – refer to the instructions on the package to determine the ideal salt-to-water ratio for your bath. <u>Follow these steps to use your Himalayan bath salts</u>:

1. Fill the tub to the desired level with very warm water (as hot as you can stand it).

2. Scoop up a handful of Himalayan bath salts (or the amount recommended on the package) and hold it under the faucet with the water running.

3. Let the salt fall into the tub where it will dissolve.

4. Climb into the tub and relax for at least 20 to 30 minutes to gain the maximum benefit from the salt.

5. Do not rinse off after your bath, simply towel yourself dry.

6. Rest for 30 minutes after drying off to allow the salt to continue soaking into your skin.

Note: The higher the concentration of Himalayan Salt in your bath water, the greater the benefits will be. Do not be afraid to add a little extra and feel free to reheat the tub with warm water as it cools.

b.) Homemade Himalayan Bath Salt Recipe

You do not necessarily need to spend a small fortune on boutique spa products to enjoy the benefits of Himalayan Salt for aging. Using this recipe, you can make your own homemade bath salts.

Ingredients:

- 3 cups coarse Himalayan Salt
- 15 to 25 drops essential oil
- 1 tablespoon jojoba oil

Instructions:

1. Place the salt in a large mixing bowl.
2. Add the jojoba oil and stir well with a wooden spoon.
3. Stir in the essential oils and mix well, then transfer the mixture to a large glass jar.
4. Seal the jar tightly and shake before using.

Notes: For this recipe you can use whatever essential oil you like – even a combination of different oils, if you prefer. Some fragrant essential oils you might consider using include lavender, rosemary, rose or eucalyptus.

2.) Himalayan Salt for Heart Health

You probably already know about the dangers of consuming too much salt in regard to heart problems. What you may not realize, however, is that these dangers apply to traditional table salt, not Himalayan Salt. Himalayan Salt is filled with 84 minerals, many of which are essential for supporting heart health. Perhaps the most important way in which Himalayan Salt supports heart health is by balancing blood pressure to prevent hypertension.

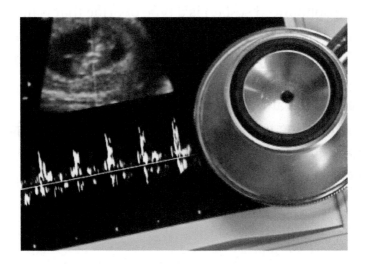

Hypertension, or high blood pressure, can be very dangerous – even fatal – but it is also easy to prevent. Himalayan Salt is completely natural which means that it is easily absorbed into your bloodstream – even a small amount of Himalayan Salt will be enough for you to experience its benefits. In regard to heart health, Himalayan Salt helps to increase circulation while also lowering blood pressure. Additionally, Himalayan Salt can help to dissolve calcified deposits in the blood vessels which can lead to a number of cardiovascular problems.

a.) Sole for Heart Health

A sole (pronounced so-lay) is a type of brine that is meant for consumption. Drinking a sole made from Himalayan Salt is a simple way to improve your heart health. To make your own sole, simply fill a glass jar about ¼ full with coarse Himalayan Salt crystals. Fill the jar the rest of the way with spring water and cover it with a lid. Let the jar rest for 24 hours then mix 1 teaspoon of the solution in a glass of water and drink it once a day before breakfast.

3.) Himalayan Salt for Brain Health

If you are familiar with the term 'pH', you may know that it refers to the measure of a substance's acidity or alkalinity on a scale from 0 to 14. You may be surprised to hear, however, that the body has a natural pH level and if that level is out of balance, it can have a severely devastating impact on your health. The human body has a naturally alkaline pH and that pH is affected by the food you eat and the beverages you drink – especially by how much water you drink.

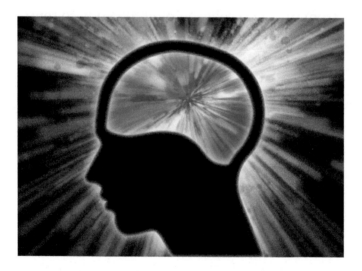

Think about it this way – the ocean is a large body of salt water with a natural pH around 8.1 (slightly alkaline like the human body). After a heavy rain storm (such as a monsoon), the added water causes the pH of the ocean to drop, making it more acidic and dangerous to the aquatic life within. In a similar way, if you drink too much water it could lead to water intoxication – this occurs when your water and sodium levels are out of balance.

So how does this relate to brain health? One important thing you should know is that the human brain is encased in water and that your brain is comprised of about 80% water. Thus, brain health is strongly linked to fluid levels in the body which are affected by sodium levels. Where Himalayan Salt comes into play is by extracting excess acidity from the brain cells, helping the body to return to its ideal pH state of alkalinity.

4.) Himalayan Salt for Bone Health

If you suffer from bone or joint issues such as arthritis and osteoporosis, your doctor may have recommended that you watch your salt intake. Common table salt can indeed contribute to the leeching of calcium from your bones which exacerbates conditions like osteoporosis, but Himalayan Salt is another story. This type of salt is all natural – in fact, it contains 84 minerals that are essential for your body. One of those minerals is calcium.

While calcium is essential for bone health and strength, supplementing your diet with too much calcium can actually be harmful. It is more beneficial to provide your body with a wide array of trace minerals, such as those found in Himalayan Salt. Osteoporosis is not just a matter of calcium loss – it is also affected by a shortage of both salt and water in the body. Incorporating Himalayan Salt in your diet is the key to maintaining fluid balance in the body and for preventing a number of serious diseases including osteoporosis.

Personal Testimony

The first time I heard about Himalayan crystal salt was 8 years ago when the wife of an acquaintance happily announced that her arthritis was gone. I was skeptical, so naturally I asked her for details. The woman's response surprised me – she said she had been taking Himalayan crystal salt. Being very interested in natural health products, I pressed the woman for more information. For years I have been experiencing soreness in my fingers and knees, though I often contributed those pains to the consequences of aging.

After speaking to the woman about Himalayan Salt, I was directed to the couple she bought it from. I spoke to this couple myself and received their very last packet of salt along with a number of informative pamphlets. I was instructed to fill a small glass with one part Himalayan salt and two parts spring water. After letting the mixture sit for 24 hours, I was to add one teaspoon of the brine to a glass of water and drink it once a day. Having nothing to lose, I gave it a try.

After a few weeks, I noticed that the soreness in my fingers and the pain in my knees had begun to dissipate. Encouraged by this development, I continued to drink my

Himalayan Salt brine each and every morning. To this day, nearly 18 months later, I am happy to say that I remain pain free – all thanks to Himalayan Salt!

5.) *Himalayan Salt for Sleep*

You may be surprised to hear it, but Himalayan Salt can actually help you to get better sleep. It can improve the quality of your sleep in two ways:

- Himalayan Salt can help to reduce your stress, calming your mind to prepare you for sleep – having adequate levels of sodium in your blood stream can actually reduce your body's stress response so you have less anxiety.

- Himalayan salt can increase your oxytocin levels – this hormone is naturally produced by the body in response to stress, helping you to feel calmer and more relaxed.

There are several ways you can use Himalayan Salt to improve your quality of sleep. One of the simplest ways is to just use Himalayan Salt to season your food throughout the day. While regular table salt can have a dehydrating effect on your body, Himalayan Salt provides a number of healthy minerals and will help you to build oxytocin levels throughout the day so you are able to relax at night when it comes time for bed.

Another great way to use Himalayan Salt to promote healthy sleep is to drink a bedtime tonic. Something as simple as a cup of chamomile tea with a dash of Himalayan Salt added can work wonders for your sleep. You might also consider taking a Himalayan Salt bath just before bed using the bath salts recipe provided earlier in this chapter. Your final option is to place a pinch of Himalayan Salt (about 1/8 teaspoon) directly on your tongue before sleep and to chase it with a small glass of water.

Chapter Six: Himalayan Salt for Cooking

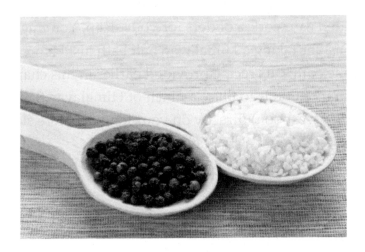

Though the majority of this book is focused on the uses of Himalayan Salt for healing, you should not forget that it can be used for a more traditional purpose as well – cooking. Himalayan Salt is still salt, after all, and it can add flavor to all of your favorite dishes. In this chapter you will learn the basics about what type of cuisine Himalayan Salt is commonly used for. You will also receive a collection of delicious recipes using Himalayan Salt in all of its forms, including salt blocks.

1.) Traditional Uses in Cuisine

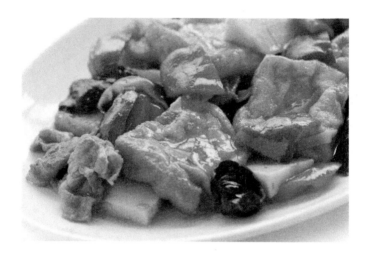

Himalayan Salt can be used in the same way as sea salt, and even table salt. Traditionally, however, it is used to preserve meats or fish – it is also a common ingredient in spice rubs and pickling brines. Earlier in this book you learned that blocks of Himalayan Salt can be slowly heated and utilized as a cooking surface for meat and seafood. In the following pages you will find a collection of recipes incorporating Himalayan Salt that you can try at home.

2.) Recipes Using Himalayan Salt

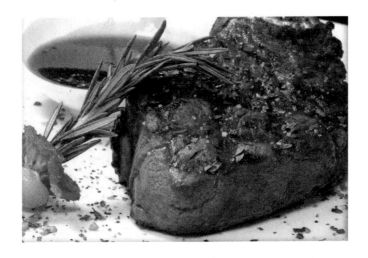

In this section you will find a variety of recipes using Himalayan Salt. <u>Recipes are divided into the following categories</u>:

Spice Rubs/Seasoning Blends

Pickling Brines

Salt Slab Recipes

Other Himalayan Salt Recipes

a.) Spice Rubs/Seasoning Blends

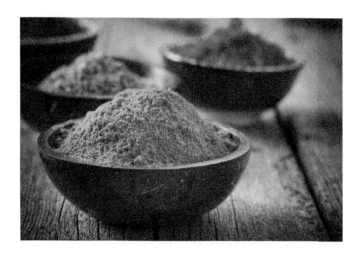

<u>Recipes Included in this Section</u>:

Spicy Dry Rub	Lemon Pepper Seasoning
Sweet Dry Rub	Seasoned Salt
Smoky Dry Rub	Fajita Seasoning
Taco Seasoning	Caribbean Jerk Seasoning
Cajun Seasoning	Asian 5-Spice Seasoning

Spicy Dry Rub

Ingredients:

- ½ cup brown sugar, packed
- ¼ cup Himalayan Salt
- ¼ cup paprika
- 3 tablespoons smoked paprika
- 2 tablespoons hot chili powder
- 3 tablespoons ground black pepper
- 1 tablespoon powdered garlic
- 1 tablespoon dried sage
- 2 teaspoons ground cumin
- 1 teaspoon cayenne powder
- ¼ teaspoon ground mace

Instructions:

1. Line a baking sheet with parchment and spread the brown sugar on the baking sheet to dry for 1 to 2 hours.
2. Transfer the sugar to a food processor and add the remaining ingredients.
3. Pulse until the mixture is well blended.
4. Store in an airtight container.
5. To use, sprinkle over meat and rub it in.
6. Wrap the meat in plastic and chill for 1 hour before cooking.

Sweet Dry Rub

Ingredients:

- ¾ cup brown sugar, packed
- ¼ cup Himalayan Salt
- ¼ cup paprika
- 2 tablespoons mild chili powder
- 2 tablespoons ground black pepper
- 1 tablespoon powdered garlic
- 1 tablespoon dried sage
- 2 teaspoons ground allspice
- 1 teaspoon ground cumin
- 1 teaspoon ground mace
- ½ teaspoon ground cloves

Instructions:

1. Line a baking sheet with parchment and spread the brown sugar on the baking sheet to dry for 1 to 2 hours.
2. Transfer the sugar to a food processor and add the remaining ingredients.
3. Pulse until the mixture is well blended.
4. Store in an airtight container.
5. To use, sprinkle over meat and rub it in.
6. Wrap the meat in plastic and chill for 1 hour before cooking.

Smoky Dry Rub

Ingredients:

- ½ cup brown sugar, packed
- ½ cup smoked paprika
- ¼ cup Himalayan Salt
- 2 tablespoons chili powder
- 2 tablespoons ground black pepper
- 1 tablespoon powdered garlic
- 1 tablespoon dried sage
- 1 teaspoon ground cumin

Instructions:

1. Line a baking sheet with parchment and spread the brown sugar on the baking sheet to dry for 1 to 2 hours.
2. Transfer the sugar to a food processor and add the remaining ingredients.
3. Pulse until the mixture is well blended.
4. Store in an airtight container.
5. To use, sprinkle over meat and rub it in.
6. Wrap the meat in plastic and chill for 1 hour before cooking.

Taco Seasoning

Ingredients:

- ¼ cup chili powder
- ¼ cup Himalayan Salt
- 3 tablespoons ground cumin
- 1 tablespoon onion powder
- 3 teaspoons garlic powder
- 1 teaspoon dried oregano
- 1 teaspoon ground black pepper
- ¾ teaspoon paprika

Instructions:

1. Combine all of the ingredients in a food processor.
2. Pulse until well blended.
3. Store the seasoning in an airtight container for up to 6 months.
4. To use, sprinkle the seasoning on ground meat and cook to brown.

Cajun Seasoning

Ingredients:

- ½ cup paprika
- ¼ cup plus 1 tablespoon Himalayan Salt
- ¼ cup powdered garlic
- 2 tablespoons onion powder
- 1 ½ tablespoons ground black pepper
- 1 tablespoon cayenne pepper
- 1 tablespoon dried oregano
- 1 tablespoon dried thyme

Instructions:

1. Combine all of the ingredients in a food processor.
2. Pulse until well blended.
3. Store the seasoning in an airtight container for up to 6 months.
4. To use, sprinkle the seasoning on poultry or eggs – can also be used in stir-fry and casseroles.

Lemon Pepper Seasoning

Ingredients:

- 5 or 6 lemons, zested
- 1/3 cup ground black pepper
- 5 tablespoons Himalayan Salt

Instructions:

1. Preheat the oven to the lowest heat setting and line a baking sheet with parchment paper.
2. Spread the lemon zest on the baking sheet and bake for 60 to 90 minutes until dried.
3. Combine the dried lemon zest with the remaining ingredients in a food processor and pulse to blend.
4. Store in an airtight container.

Seasoned Salt

Ingredients:

- ½ cup Himalayan Salt
- ¼ cup onion powder
- ¼ cup powdered garlic
- ¼ cup ground black pepper
- 2 tablespoons chili powder
- 2 tablespoons paprika

Instructions:

1. Combine all of the ingredients in a food processor.
2. Pulse until well blended.
3. Store the seasoning in an airtight container for up to 6 months.

Fajita Seasoning

Ingredients:

- ¼ cup chili powder
- 2 tablespoons Himalayan Salt
- 2 tablespoons paprika
- 1 tablespoon powdered garlic
- 1 tablespoon ground cumin
- 3 teaspoons onion powder
- 2 teaspoons cayenne powder

Instructions:

1. Combine all of the ingredients in a food processor.
2. Pulse until well blended.
3. Store the seasoning in an airtight container for up to 6 months.
4. To use, sprinkle the seasoning on sliced chicken or beef and cook to brown.

Caribbean Jerk Seasoning

Ingredients:

- ¼ cup onion powder
- 2 tablespoons Himalayan Salt
- 2 tablespoons ground thyme
- 1 tablespoon ground cinnamon
- ½ tablespoon ground allspice
- 1 to 2 teaspoons cayenne powder

Instructions:

1. Combine all of the ingredients in a food processor.
2. Pulse until well blended.
3. Store the seasoning in an airtight container for up to 6 months.

Asian 5-Spice Seasoning

Ingredients:

- ¼ cup anise powder
- 2 tablespoons ground black pepper
- 2 tablespoons Himalayan Salt
- 2 tablespoons ground cinnamon
- 2 tablespoons ground fennel
- 1 tablespoon ground cloves

Instructions:

1. Combine all of the ingredients in a food processor.
2. Pulse until well blended.
3. Store the seasoning in an airtight container for up to 6 months.
4. Use in stir-fries and other Asian-style recipes.

b.) Pickling Brines

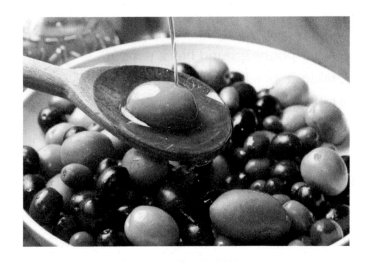

Recipes Included in this Section:

Basic Pickling Brine

Orange-Spiced Beets

Dill Pickles

Old-Fashioned Sauerkraut

Pickled Green Beans

Herbed Carrot Sticks

Basic Himalayan Salt Pickling Brine

In order to pickle vegetables, you will need a basic pickling brine – a 2% brine is ideal for firm vegetables like carrots, beets, and beans. Pickling cucumbers may require a higher salinity, however, between 3.5% and 5%.

2% Brine

Ingredients:

- 2 quarts (8 cups) water
- 2 ½ tablespoons Himalayan Salt

Instructions:

1. Fill a large pitcher with 2 quarts of water.
2. Stir in the salt and let it sit for at least 1 hour.

3.5% Brine

- 2 quarts (8 cups) water
- 4 ½ tablespoons Himalayan Salt

5% Brine

- 2 quarts (8 cups) water
- 6 tablespoons plus 1 teaspoon Himalayan Salt

Orange-Spiced Beets

Ingredients:

- 8 medium beets
- 1 (3-inch) stick cinnamon
- 1 inch fresh ginger
- 4 whole cloves
- 1 teaspoon allspice berries
- 1 teaspoon mustard seeds
- 1 teaspoon whole peppercorns
- 1 teaspoon cardamom seeds
- 2 to 3 tablespoons orange zest
- ¼ cup fresh orange juice
- 2% brine

Instructions:

1. Combine all of the ingredients except for the beets and the brine in a 1-gallon jar.
2. Scrub the beets well then cut off the roots and top.
3. Chop the beets into 1-inch cubes then add them to the jar.
4. Fill the jar the rest of the way with 2% brine, stopping just below the neck of the jar.
5. Seal the jar with a lid and let sit for 7 to 9 days.
6. Refrigerate the jar after opening.

Dill Pickles

Ingredients:

- Pickling cucumbers, freshly picked
- 3 heads garlic, cloves separated and peeled
- 5 sprigs fresh dill
- 1 ½ tablespoons coriander seeds
- 1 teaspoon whole cloves
- 1 teaspoon whole mustard seed
- 1 teaspoon whole peppercorns
- 1 teaspoon fennel seeds
- 1-inch cinnamon stick
- 2 grape leaves
- 3.5% or 5% brine

Instructions:

1. Wash the pickles and trim off the ends.
2. Combine the herbs and spices in a 1 ½ gallon jar.
3. Pack in the cucumbers, making sure they stand vertically in the jar – stuff them in tight.
4. Pour in the brine to fill the jar just below the neck – 3.5% brine will yield half-sour pickles, 5% brine full sour.
5. Tightly cover the jar with a lid and store in a cool area for 7 to 12 days.
6. Refrigerate after opening.

Old-Fashioned Sauerkraut

Ingredients:

- 4 lbs. sliced green cabbage
- 4 teaspoons Himalayan Salt
- 2% brine

Instructions:

1. Toss the sliced cabbage with Himalayan Salt in a large mixing bowl.
2. Pack the cabbage into a 1-gallon jar, pressing it against the sides to release any liquid.
3. Let the cabbage sit for 1 hour.
4. Fill the jar to just below the neck with brine.
5. Cover the jar tightly with a lid and let sit in a 70°F area for 8 to 10 days.
6. Move to cool storage and store for at least 6 weeks before using.
7. Refrigerate the jar after opening.

Note: You may also add up to 2 teaspoons of whole caraway seed to season the cabbage when you toss it with the Himalayan Salt.

Pickled Green Beans

Ingredients:

- Green beans, freshly picked
- 2 medium sprigs rosemary
- 2% pickling brine

Instructions:

1. Trim the ends off the beans and remove any soft spots or blemishes.
2. Combine the herbs in the bottom of a 1-gallon jar.
3. Pack in the beans vertically, stuffing in as many as you possibly can.
4. Pour in the brine, filling the jar to just below the neck.
5. Store at 70°F for 7 to 10 days.
6. Move the jar to the refrigerator and enjoy once chilled.

Note: You may also use fresh basil or dill as a substitute for the rosemary in this recipe.

Herbed Carrot Sticks

Ingredients:

- Fresh carrots (about 2 lbs.)
- 1 sprig fresh dill
- 2% pickling brine

Instructions:

1. Place the dill in the bottom of a 1-gallon jar.
2. Pack the jar with carrots, filling it to the neck of the jar.
3. Pour in the brine to fill the jar to the neck.
4. Cover tightly with a lid and leave at room temperature for 7 to 9 days.
5. Transfer the jar to the refrigerator and store for 2 to 3 weeks before enjoying.

Note: There are several ways you can prepare the carrots for this recipe. It is recommended that you slice them lengthwise, though you can trim the pieces as small as you like. You can also use grated carrots. You may also substitute other herbs for the dill – try mint or ginger.

c.) Salt Slab Recipes

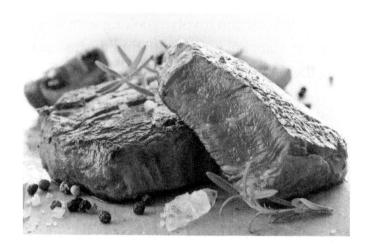

<u>Recipes Included in this Section</u>:

Scallops with Garlic and Olive Oil

Cilantro Lime Shrimp

Seared Flank Steak

Rosemary Shrimp Skewers

Mahi Mahi with Coconut Rum

Chilean Sea Bass

Garlic Grilled Chicken

Chilled Melon and Feta

Heating a Salt Block on the Stove

The recipes in this section involve cooking with a
Himalayan Salt slab. Below you will find the instructions
for heating the slab:

1. Select a salt slab at least 1.5 to 2 inches thick.

2. Place the block directly on the grate over a gas grill
   or on the burner of a gas stove.

3. For an electric stove, place a metal ring around the
   burner to keep the block from resting directly on it.

4. Turn the burner or grill on to the lowest heat setting
   and let the block heat for 15 minutes – it should reach
   about 200°F.

5. Increase the heat to medium and let the block heat
   for another 10 minutes.

6. Turn up the heat to high and let the block heat for
   another 10 minutes until it is fully heated.

7. If your block is more than 2 inches thick or wider
   than 8 inches, it could take longer to heat.

Scallops with Garlic and Olive Oil

Ingredients:

- 1 lbs. raw sea scallops
- 2 tablespoons olive oil
- 1 tablespoon minced garlic

Instructions:

1. Preheat the salt slab to about 400°F.
2. Combine the olive oil and garlic in a small bowl.
3. Rinse the scallops in cool water then pat dry with paper towel.
4. Brush the scallops with the olive oil and garlic blend.
5. Place the scallops on the preheated salt slab.
6. Cook for 2 to 3 minutes to sear the scallops on one side then carefully flip them over.
7. Sear the scallops on the other side until just cooked through.

Cilantro Lime Shrimp

Ingredients:

- 2 lbs. uncooked shrimp, peeled and deveined
- 2 to 3 ripe limes, halved
- 2 tablespoons olive oil
- 1 cup fresh chopped cilantro

Instructions:

1. Preheat the salt slab to about 400°F.
2. Squeeze the lime onto the shrimp and toss well to coat.
3. Let the shrimp rest for 15 minutes.
4. Drizzle the olive oil onto the preheated salt slab and arrange the shrimp on it in a single layer.
5. Cook the shrimp for 2 to 3 minutes on each side until pink and firm.
6. Toss the shrimp with cilantro to serve.

Seared Flank Steak

Ingredients:

1 lbs. boneless flank steak

Instructions:

1. Preheat the salt slab to about 400°F.
2. Slice the flank steak with the grain of the meat into thin slices – about ¼ to ½ inch thick.
3. Arrange the slices on the preheated salt slab.
4. Cook for 20 to 30 seconds on one side until lightly browned.
5. Carefully flip the steak strips and brown on the other side.
6. If you prefer your steak well-done, the cooking time may be longer.

Rosemary Shrimp Skewers

Ingredients:

- 2 lbs. uncooked shrimp, peeled and deveined
- 1 tablespoon olive oil
- 6 to 8 long sprigs fresh rosemary
- 2 tablespoons chopped garlic

Instructions:

1. Preheat the salt slab to about 400°F.
2. Strip the leaves from the rosemary sprigs, leaving the woody stem.
3. Slide the shrimp onto the rosemary stems, using them as skewers.
4. Drizzle the olive oil over the preheated salt slab.
5. Lay the shrimp skewers flat on the slab and sprinkle with chopped garlic.
6. Cook the shrimp for 2 to 3 minutes then flip and sprinkle the other side with garlic.
7. Let the shrimp cook for another 2 minutes or so until pink and firm.

Mahi Mahi with Coconut Rum

Ingredients:

- 4 (5 to 6 ounce) mahi mahi fillets, boneless
- ¼ cup coconut rum
- 1 tablespoon olive oil

Instructions:

1. Preheat the salt slab to about 400°F.
2. Place the fillets in a shallow glass container and pour the coconut rum over them.
3. Let the fillets rest for 15 minutes to absorb the rum.
4. Drizzle the olive oil over the preheated salt slab.
5. Place the fillets on the slab and cook for 2 to 3 minutes on each side to sear.

Chilean Sea Bass

Ingredients:

- 4 (4 to 5 ounce) Chilean sea bass fillets
- 1 tablespoon olive oil
- Thinly sliced lemon

Instructions:

1. Preheat the salt slab to about 400°F.
2. Drizzle the olive oil on the preheated salt slab.
3. Place the fillets on the slab and cook for 2 to 3 minutes until just seared.
4. Flip the fillets and top with lemon slices.
5. Cook for another 2 to 3 minutes until seared, or cooked to the desired level.
6. Serve the fillets hot with extra lemon.

Garlic Grilled Chicken

Ingredients:

- 4 chicken leg quarters
- 2 tablespoons olive oil
- 1 tablespoon chopped garlic
- Freshly ground black pepper

Instructions:

1. Preheat a salt block on a grill to about 400°F.
2. Rinse the chicken leg quarters in cool water and pat it dry.
3. Rub the chicken with olive oil and garlic and season with ground pepper.
4. Remove the salt block from the grill and place the chicken leg quarters on the grill, skin side down.
5. Place the salt block on top of the chicken and cook for 15 minutes with the lid closed.
6. Flip the chicken, placing the salt blocks back on top, and cook for another 10 to 15 minutes until the chicken reaches an internal temperature of 170°F.
7. Remove the salt blocks and let the chicken rest on a cutting board for 5 minutes before serving.

Chilled Melon and Feta

Ingredients:

- ½ small watermelon, peel removed and sliced
- ½ small cantaloupe, peel removed and sliced
- ½ cup crumbled feta cheese
- Fresh mint leaves, coarsely chopped

Instructions:

1. Place a salt slab in the refrigerator to chill for at least 2 hours.
2. Remove the slab from the refrigerator and arrange the melon slices on top of it.
3. Arrange the melon slices to that they are slightly overlapping so they do not absorb too much salt.
4. Sprinkle the melon slices with feta and mint leaves.
5. Serve immediately or, for more flavor, let the melon rest on the slab for 15 to 20 minutes first.

d.) Other Himalayan Salt Recipes

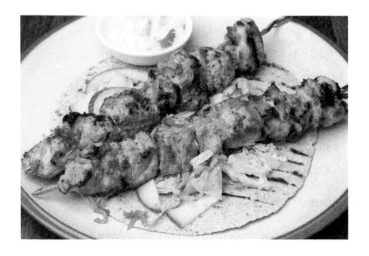

<u>Recipes Included in this Section</u>:

Salted Rosemary Bread	Salmon with Pear Puree
Chopped Shrimp Salad	Salted Chocolate Cupcakes
Sautéed Beet Greens	Chocolate Chip Cookies
Tomato Mozzarella Salad	Salted Butter Caramels
Grape Almond Gazpacho	Salty Dog Cocktail

Salted Rosemary Bread

Ingredients:

- ¾ cup sourdough starter
- 2 cups warm water
- 3 cups all-purpose flour
- 1 cup whole-wheat flour
- ¾ tablespoon coarse Himalayan Salt
- ¼ cup fresh chopped rosemary
- ¼ cup fresh chopped garlic

Instructions:

1. Place the sourdough starter in a large mixing bowl.
2. Stir in the water, whole-wheat flour and all-purpose flour then let rest for 20 minutes.
3. Work the salt into the dough then cover with a clean towel and set in a warm place to rise for 2 to 3 hours.
4. Place a Dutch oven inside the oven and preheat the oven to 450°F.
5. Turn the dough out onto a floured surface and knead it several times.
6. Pat the dough flat into a thick circle by hand and sprinkle with rosemary and garlic.
7. Fold the sides of the dough in then roll the dough into a loose ball and pinch the sides together.
8. Use a sharp knife to cut several lines across the surface of the dough – the lines should not be more than a few millimeters thick.

9. Place the loaf inside the preheated Dutch oven and cover with the lid.
10. Bake for 30 minutes then remove the lid and lower the oven temperature to 400°F.
11. Let the bread bake for another 10 to 15 minutes, then remove from the oven and let it rest for 1 hour.
12. Make sure the bread is cool before slicing it.

Chopped Shrimp Salad

Ingredients:

- ½ lbs. cooked shrimp, thawed
- Himalayan Salt to taste
- ¼ cup olive oil
- 3 tablespoons fresh lime juice
- ¼ cup fresh chopped cilantro
- 5 cups chopped romaine lettuce
- 1 cup thinly sliced red cabbage
- 2 green onions, thinly sliced

Instructions:

1. Rinse the shrimp in cool water then pat dry with paper towel.
2. Combine the olive oil, lime juice and cilantro in a food processor and blend until smooth.
3. Place the shrimp in a mixing bowl and sprinkle with Himalayan Salt.
4. Toss the shrimp with 2 to 3 tablespoons of the dressing and set aside to marinate.
5. Combine the romaine, cabbage, and green onions in a salad bowl.
6. Toss with the dressed shrimp and the remaining dressing to serve.

Sautéed Beet Greens

Ingredients:

- 1 large bunch fresh beet greens
- 1 tablespoon olive oil
- ½ tablespoon minced garlic
- 1 shallot, diced
- 2 teaspoons white sugar
- ¼ teaspoon Himalayan Salt
- ½ teaspoon freshly ground pepper
- ¼ cup water
- 2 teaspoons red wine vinegar

Instructions:

1. Rinse the beet greens well then trim the stems.
2. Heat the oil in a large skillet over medium heat.
3. Add the garlic and shallot and cook for 2 minutes until fragrant.
4. Stir in the sugar, Himalayan Salt and pepper.
5. Add the beet greens and pour the water over them.
6. Cover the skillet immediately and cook for 1 to 2 minutes until the greens have cooked down.
7. Stir the greens and cook, uncovered, for another 1 to 2 minutes until the water evaporates.
8. Drizzle with vinegar to serve.

Tomato, Basil, Mozzarella Salad

Ingredients:

- 1 ball fresh mozzarella
- 2 medium ripe tomatoes, sliced
- ½ cup fresh chopped basil
- Himalayan Salt
- Freshly ground pepper

Instructions:

1. Slice the fresh mozzarella into thin slices, no more than ¼-inch thick.
2. Alternate the tomato and mozzarella slices on a serving platter.
3. Season the tomato and mozzarella with Himalayan Salt and freshly ground pepper.
4. Drizzle with balsamic vinegar then sprinkle with chopped basil to serve.

Grape Almond Gazpacho

Ingredients:

- 2 cups blanched almonds
- 3 tablespoons chopped garlic
- 3 cups water
- 1 cup white grape juice
- 3 ounces sherry vinegar
- 1 cup extra-virgin olive oil
- Himalayan Salt to taste
- Freshly ground pepper
- Ripe grapes

Instructions:

1. Soak the almonds in water overnight then rinse well and drain.
2. Combine the almonds with the garlic, water, grape juice and sherry vinegar in a food processor.
3. Blend until smooth and well combined.
4. With the processor running, drizzle in the olive oil.
5. Season with Himalayan Salt and freshly ground pepper to taste then cover and chill for several hours.
6. Spoon into small bowls and garnish with fresh grapes to serve.

Salmon with Pear Puree

Ingredients:

- 4 (6-ounce) boneless salmon fillets
- 2 ripe Bartlett pears
- ½ teaspoon fresh minced ginger
- 1 ½ tablespoons olive oil
- ¼ cup dry white wine
- 1 cup fresh spinach, packed
- Himalayan Salt to taste
- Freshly ground pepper

Instructions:

1. Bring a pot of water to boil and add the pears.
2. Blanch the pears for 30 second then plunge into ice water and drain well.
3. Chop the pears and puree them in a food processor with the ginger.
4. Transfer the mixture to a small saucepan and warm over medium heat.
5. Heat the oil in a large skillet over medium-high heat.
6. Add the salmon fillets and cook for 2 minutes on each side until lightly browned.
7. Pour in the white wine then add the spinach and sprinkle with Himalayan Salt and fresh pepper.
8. Cover the skillet and cook for 2 to 3 minutes until the salmon is cooked through.

9. Spoon some of the pear puree onto each of four plates and top with a salmon fillet and some of the spinach to serve.

Salted Chocolate Cupcakes

Ingredients:

- 2 cups cake flour
- ½ cup unsweetened cocoa powder
- 2 teaspoons baking powder
- 1 teaspoon baking soda
- ¼ teaspoon kosher salt
- 1 ½ cups white sugar
- 1 cup mayonnaise
- 1 ½ cups water
- 1 teaspoon vanilla extract
- 1 cup heavy cream
- 14 ounces dark chocolate, chopped
- Coarse Himalayan Salt

Instructions:

1. Preheat the oven to 350°F and line a muffin pan with paper liners.
2. Combine the cake flour, cocoa powder, baking powder, baking soda and kosher salt in a large mixing bowl and stir well.
3. In a separate bowl, whisk together the sugar, mayonnaise and vanilla extract.
4. Add about ⅓ of the flour mixture to the mayonnaise and whisk well.
5. Whisk in ½ of the water then repeat, alternating between adding the dry ingredients and water and whisking between each addition.

6. Beat the mixture for 2 minutes until light and airy.
7. Spoon the batter into the prepared pan, filling each cup about 2/3 full.
8. Bake the cupcakes for 18 to 25 minutes until a knife inserted in the center comes out clean.
9. Set the cupcakes aside to cool while you prepare the ganache.
10. Heat the cream in a small saucepan over medium-low heat – do not boil.
11. Place the chopped chocolate in a heat-proof bowl and pour the hot cream over it.
12. Let the chocolate sit for 1 minute then stir well.
13. Transfer the bowl to the refrigerator and chill, stirring occasionally, until it thickens.
14. Spoon the ganache into a piping bag and pipe it onto the cooled cupcakes.
15. Sprinkle with Himalayan Salt and serve.

Salted Chocolate Chip Cookies

Ingredients:

- 1 ½ cups all-purpose flour
- 1 teaspoon baking powder
- ¼ teaspoon baking soda
- ½ teaspoon kosher salt
- 1 stick unsalted butter, softened
- ¾ cup brown sugar, packed
- ¾ cup granulated white sugar
- 1 large egg plus 2 yolks
- 1 teaspoon vanilla extract
- 1 ½ cups semisweet chocolate chips
- Himalayan Salt to taste

Instructions:

1. Preheat the oven to 375°F.
2. Combine the flour, baking powder, baking soda and kosher salt in a mixing bowl.
3. In a separate bowl, beat the butter and sugars on high speed until light and fluffy.
4. Add the eggs and vanilla and beat until smooth.
5. In small batches, add the dry ingredients and beat until just combined.
6. Fold in the chocolate chips then drop the batter in 1-inch balls onto parchment-lined baking sheet.
7. Sprinkle the balls of dough with Himalayan Salt then bake for 10 to 12 minutes, turning halfway through.

8. Cool the cookies for 3 to 4 minutes on the baking sheets then transfer to wire racks to cool completely.

Salted Butter Caramels

Ingredients:

- 3 cups heavy cream
- 1 cup unsalted butter, chopped
- ½ teaspoon kosher salt
- 3 cups granulated white sugar
- 1 cup light corn syrup
- 1 ¼ teaspoons vanilla extract
- Himalayan Salt to taste

Instructions:

1. Line a large rectangular glass baking dish with parchment paper and grease with cooking spray.
2. Combine the cream, butter and kosher salt in a small saucepan over medium heat.
3. Bring the mixture to a simmer while whisking then remove from heat.
4. In a deep stockpot, combine the sugar and corn syrup.
5. Bring to a boil and swirl the pot (do not stir) until the mixture turns golden brown.
6. Turn off the heat and slowly pour in the cream mixture.
7. Use a wooden spoon to stir in the vanilla extract.
8. Boil over medium-low heat for another 20 to 30 minutes until it reaches 248°F on a candy thermometer – only stir once in a while to keep it from sticking.

9. Pour the mixture into the prepared dish and chill for 30 to 60 minutes until firm.
10. Turn out the caramel onto a cutting board and remove the parchment paper.
11. Coat a sharp knife with oil and cut the caramel into four long pieces.
12. Cut the long pieces into thin slices and sprinkle lightly with Himalayan Salt.
13. Wrap the caramels individually in pieces of parchment paper to serve.
14. Store in an airtight container in the refrigerator.

Salty Dog Cocktail

Ingredients:

- medium-grain Himalayan Salt
- 1 grapefruit wedge
- ½ cup fresh grapefruit juice
- 1 ounce vodka
- 1 tablespoon grenadine
- ½ to 1 cup ice cubes

Instructions:

1. Pour some medium-grain Himalayan Salt into a shallow dish.
2. Moisten the rim of a cocktail glass with the grapefruit wedge then dip it in the salt.
3. Combine the grapefruit juice, vodka and grenadine in a blender.
4. Blend for 10 seconds on high speed.
5. With the blender running, drop in the ice cubes and blend until smooth.
6. Pour the beverage into the rimmed glass to serve.

Chapter Seven: The Truth about Table Salt

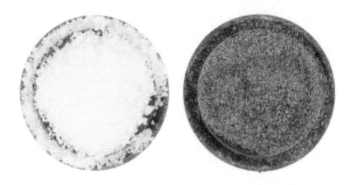

When you think of the term "salt", you probably picture a cylindrical cardboard canister filled with tiny white crystals – you may also picture a glass shaker sitting on your kitchen table. While table salt is incredibly common, many people do not realize that is also incredibly dangerous. In this chapter you will learn the hazards that traditional table salt poses to your health and why Himalayan Salt is better. By the time you finish this chapter you will be ready to toss your table salt over your shoulder and straight into the trash can.

1.) Where Table Salt Comes From

What you know as "table salt" is a commercially manufactured form of sodium, called sodium chloride. This chemical is similar in taste to naturally-occurring salts like Himalayan Salt and sea salt, but that is where the comparisons end. Table salt is made by cooking natural salt at extremely high temperatures, around 1200°F to remove impurities. In the process, however, most of the natural mineral content of the salt is lost as well – this includes the trace elements that are essential for keeping the body hydrated and fluid levels balanced.

After the salt is chemically cleaned, it is often "refined" with synthetic chemicals. <u>Some of the chemicals commonly added to table salt include</u>:

- Solo-co-aluminate
- Iodide
- Sodium bicarbonate
- Fluoride
- Anti-caking agents
- Potassium iodide
- Aluminum derivatives

You may notice that iodide is often added to table salt. If you think back to the earlier chapters of this book, you may remember that iodine is an important natural element in salt that supports the thyroid. During processing, however, much of the natural iodine content is lost so manufacturers add synthetic iodide to table salt to take its place. Unfortunately, this synthetic form of iodine can severely damage the thyroid which may lead to issues with growth and metabolism.

Another thing you should think about in regard to table salt is its color. By now you should know that natural salt, particularly Himalayan Salt, is not pure white. So how does table salt get its bright-white color? The answer is simple – manufacturers add bleach to color the salt. Other additives like anti-caking agents and MSG are also commonly used in processing table salt.

2.) Dangers of Table Salt

While earlier in this book you learned that salt is essential for proper health, it is important to realize that there are different types of salt and not all of them are good for you. Table salt, for example, has been chemically "cleaned", having most of its naturally mineral content removed and replaced with synthetic chemicals. You may be shocked to hear that the minerals stripped from salt to create table salt are often then sold to supplement companies. This means that the manufacturers producing table salt understand the benefit of the minerals they are removing but they continue to make a product that can be harmful to your body.

So, how exactly does table salt harm your body?

- In the absence of vital minerals, table salt causes fluctuations in blood pressure rather than helping to stabilize it

- Contains inadequate amounts of iodine to prevent/compensate for iodine deficiencies

- Toxic additives like ferrocyanide, talc and silica aluminate are used to make table salt flow more easily

- o Aluminum intake is particularly linked to neurological disorders

- o Talc is known to be a carcinogen, though further tests on its effects are needed

- o Aluminum bioaccumulates in the body, increasing its degenerative effects over time

- Your body expends tremendous amounts of energy to metabolize table salt crystals

- Inorganic forms of sodium can upset the fluid balance in your body

- Water is drawn out of your cells to break up and neutralize sodium chloride particles, resulting in dehydrated cells and premature cell death

  - o For each gram of sodium chloride your body can't excrete, it uses 23 times the amount of cellular water to neutralize it

- Fluoride, another common additive for table salt, has been shown to interfere with the function of nerve cells in the brain

o   Fluoride may also increase manganese absorption
    in the body – manganese is also linked to
    cognitive problems

So why do people still use salt? The answer is simple –
manufacturing companies use targeted advertising
campaigns to convince consumers that additives like iodine
and fluoride are healthy.

a.) What About Low-Sodium Foods?

Given the dangers of consuming processed foods with a
high sodium content, you may be tempted to switch to
some of the low-sodium options that have started to appear
on the market. These products are targeted toward
customers who are concerned about their daily sodium
intake but prey on their naiveté.

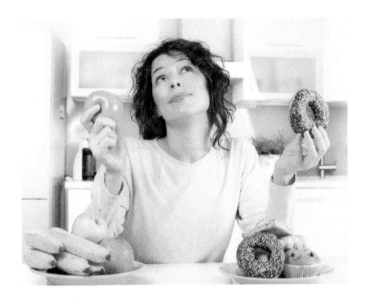

While these products may be comparatively low in sodium
chloride (table salt), they are often high in monosodium
glutamate, a sodium-based excitotoxin that has been linked
to severe health problems, namely heart attacks in
individuals with low magnesium levels. Low-sodium foods

are particularly dangerous for athletes who lose a significant portion of their natural sodium and electrolytes through sweating – the addition of monosodium glutamate then adds to that problem by causing further imbalance.

3.) Why Himalayan Salt is Better

After reading about the dangers of traditional table salt, you may have already made the decision to eliminate it from your household. In this section, however, you will learn what makes Himalayan Salt a better option, referencing the specific dangers posed by table salt.

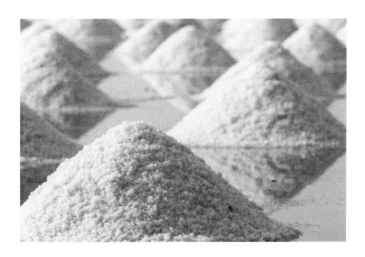

The first thing you need to realize is that Himalayan Salt is completely natural – it is unrefined, which means that its mineral content is unaltered (think back to how table salt is chemically "cleaned" to remove impurities, and thus its natural mineral content). One of the 84 minerals Himalayan Salt naturally contains is iodine – not that synthetic form called iodide. Iodine is an essential mineral that the body needs to produce the thyroid hormones that are needed to regulate the metabolism and to support healthy growth. The synthetic iodide in table salt can actually hamper the thyroid, impairing these functions.

If you paid attention during the introductory chapters of this book, you already know that Himalayan Salt is an ancient substance – it is over 250 million years old. Additionally, Himalayan Salt is completely pure and natural which means that it doesn't contain toxic additives like ferrocyanide, talc and silica aluminate that are used in table salt. It is also worth noting that Himalayan Salt crystals are stable and safe for consumption – each molecule is interconnected through molecular vibrations. Table salt crystals, on the other hand, are often treated like foreign invaders in the body (due to chemical alterations) and it takes a vast amount of energy to neutralize them.

Chapter Eight: Relevant Websites

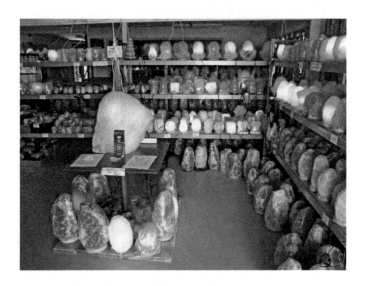

After reading this book, you should be convinced of the merits of Himalayan Salt – you may even be ready to start experiencing some of its benefits for yourself. If you are, this chapter is the perfect place to start. Here you will find a collection of websites and other resources where you can purchase Himalayan Salt and learn more about it.

1.) United States Websites

Salt Works – Gourmet Himalayan Salt.

<http://www.saltworks.us/himalayan-salt.asp#.U8Qq_vldXX4>

Mountain Rose Herbs – Kosher Himalayan Pink Salt.

<https://www.mountainroseherbs.com/products/himalayan-pink-salt/profile>

Tropical Traditions – Himalayan Pink Salt.

<http://www.tropicaltraditions.com/himalayan_salt.htm>

HimalaSalt – The Purest Salt on Earth.

<http://www.himalasalt.com/>

The Meadow – Himalayan Pink Salt Blocks, Plates, Platters & Bowls.

<http://www.atthemeadow.com/shop/Gourmet-Sea-Salt/Himalayan-Salt-Blocks>

2.) United Kingdom Websites

Cult Beauty – Himalayan Detox Salts.

<http://www.cultbeauty.co.uk/therapie-himalayan-detox-salts.html>

Salty Lamps – Himalayan Salt Lamps.

<http://www.saltylamps.co.uk/>

Himalayan Crystal Salt – Himalayan Salt.

<http://www.himalayancrystalsalt.co.uk/home.asp>

Bobby's Health Shop – Himalayan Crystal Salt.

<http://www.bobbyshealthyshop.co.uk/Himalayan-Salts.php>

WestLab – Himalayan Pink Salt Bath and Food Grade.

<http://www.westlab.co.uk/himalayan-pink-salt-25kg>

3.) Australian Websites

Himalayan Salt Factory – Shopping and Retail.

<https://www.facebook.com/pages/Himalayan-Salt-factory/432879286842480>

SafeSalt - Holistic Himalayan Salt.

<http://www.safesalt.com.au/>

Rock Salt Lamps.

<http://www.rocksaltlamps.com.au/>

Perfect Health – Himalayan Rock Salt Lamps.

<http://www.perfecthealthnow.com.au/products/himalayan
-salt-products/rock-salt-lamps/>

References

"A Brief History of Salt." Real Salt. <http://realsalt.com/sea-salt/a-brief-history-of-salt/>

"Alkalizing 101: Salt and Vibrant Health." The Chalk Board. <http://thechalkboardmag.com/alkalizing-101-the-truth-about-salt-for-your-health>

Annigan, Jan. "The Relationships Between Salt & Potassium." SF Gate. <http://healthyeating.sfgate.com/relationships-between-salt-potassium-6609.html>

"Aromatherapy Bath Salts Recipe." AromaWeb. <http://www.aromaweb.com/recipes/bathsalts.asp>

"Chemical Analysis of Natural Himalayan Pink Rock Salt." SaltNews.com. <http://www.saltnews.com/chemical-analysis-natural-himalayan-pink-salt/>

Corriher, C. Thomas. "The Truth About Table Salt and the Chemical Industry." The Healthy Wyze Report.

<http://healthwyze.org/index.php/component/content/articl
e/115-the-truth-about-table-salt-and-the-chemical-
industry.html>

"Guide to Curing with Salt." The Meadow.
<http://www.atthemeadow.com/shop/Resources/Guide-to-
Curing-with-Salt>

"HimalaSalt – HimalaSalt's Ancient Story, Himalayan Pink
Salt from the Himalayas." HimalaSalt.com.
<http://www.himalasalt.com/index.php?page=product&dis
play=8>

"Himalayan Salt Lamps." Mercola.com.
<http://products.mercola.com/himalayan-salt/himalayan-
salt-lamps.htm>

"Himalayan Salt – The Benefits for You." Life Begins Raw.
<http://www.lifebeginsraw.com/himalayan_salt_-
_the_benefits_for_you.html>

Holden, Maryann. "Balancing Effect of Himalayan Crystal
Salt on Blood Pressure and Heart Circulatory Diseases."
Boomer Living. <http://www.boomer-

livingplus.com/article/balancing_effect_of_himalayan_cryst
al_salt_on_blood_pressure_and_heart_circ>

"How Salt Can Help You Get Better Sleep." Healy Eats
Real. <http://healyeatsreal.com/how-salt-can-help-you-get-
better-sleep/>

"How to Cook Steak on a Himalayan Salt Block." The
Meadow. <http://www.atthemeadow.com/shop/resources/
cook-steak-on-himalayan-salt-block>

"How to Use Bath Salts." San Francisco Salt Company.
<http://www.bathsalt.net/How_to_Use_Bath_Salts.html>

"Iodine." The World's Healthiest Foods.
<http://www.whfoods.com/genpage.php?tname=nutrient&
dbid=69>

Mercola, Dr. Joseph. "How to Use Himalayan Salt Crystals
for Healing." Food Matters.
<http://www.foodmatters.tv/articles-1/how-to-use-
himalayan-salt-crystals-for-healing>

"Minerals in Himalayan Pink Salt – Spectral Analysis." The Meadow. <http://www.atthemeadow.com/shop/resources/minerals-in-pink-himalayan-salt>

"Real Salt, Celtic Salt and Himalayan Salt." Dr. Sircus.com. <http://drsircus.com/medicine/salt/real-salt-celtic-salt-and-himalayan-salt>

"Salt Information." SaltWorks.com. <http://www.saltworks.us/himalayan-salt.asp#.U6BnyPldXX4>

"Sea Salt vs. Table Salt. Does it Really Matter?" Chris Beat Cancer. <http://www.chrisbeatcancer.com/salt-not-the-movie-the-mineral/>

"Table Salt is Poison." Healing Naturally by Bee. <http://www.healingnaturallybybee.com/articles/salt6.php>

"Table Salt Versus Himalayan Salt." XBrain. <http://www.xbrain.co.uk/table-salt-versus-himalayan-salt>

"The Benefits of Himalayan Salt." Global Healing Center. <http://www.globalhealingcenter.com/natural-health/himalayan-crystal-salt-benefits/>

"The Health Dangers of Salt." Global Healing Center. <http://www.globalhealingcenter.com/natural-health/dangers-of-salt/>

"The Many Benefits of Himalayan Crystal Bath Salts." Mercola.com. <http://products.mercola.com/himalayan-salt/bath-salt.htm>

"What is Himalayan Salt?" YourSaltLamps.com. <http://www.yoursaltlamps.com/faq.php>

"What is Magnesium? How it Functions in the Body." Ancient Minerals. <http://www.ancient-minerals.com/magnesium-benefits/what-is-function/>

Photo Credits

Cover Page Photo By Bad Soden Salzgrotte (salt therapy room), By Reise-Line via Wikimedia Commons, <http://en.wikipedia.org/wiki/ File:Bad_Soden_Salzgrotte.JPG>

Page 1 Photo By Rainer Z via Wikimedia Commons, <http://en.wikipedia.org/wikarrisoni/File:Himalaya-Salz-1.jpg>

Page 5 Photo By NASA via Wikimedia Commons, <http://commons.wikimedia.org/wiki/Himalayas#mediavie wer/File:Himalayas.jpg>

Page 7 Photo By Bernard Gagnon via Wikimedia Commons, http://en.wikipedia.org/wiki/ File:Dead_Sea,_Jordan_02.jpg

Page 11 Photo By Khewra Salt Mine, By Shikari7 via Wikimedia Commons, <http://en.wikipedia.org/wiki/File:Khewra_Salt_Mine_-_Crystal_Deposits_on_the_mine_walls.jpg>

Page 13 Photo By Farhan, via Wikimedia Commons, <http://en.wikipedia.org/wiki/File:Khewra_Salt_Mines_Paki stan_(206).jpg>

Page 15 Photo Purchased from BigStockPhoto.net

Page 17 Photo By Dawoodmajoka via Wikimedia Commons, <http://en.wikipedia.org/wiki/ File:SaltLamps.JPG>

Page 20 Photo By Lordtct via Wikimedia Commons, <http://en.wikipedia.org/wiki/Himalayan_salt#mediaviewer /File:Himalayan_Rock_Salt.jpg>

Page 23 Photo By Sushant salva via Wikimedia Commons, <http://en.wikipedia.org/wiki/ Himalayan_salt#mediaviewer/File:Himalayan_Rock_Salt.jp g>

Page 25 Photo By Jellyboots via Wikimedia Commons, <http://en.wikipedia.org/wiki/Himalayan_salt#mediaviewer /File:Himalayan_Rock_Salt.jpg>

Page 28 Photo By DeadSeaIsrael5 via Wikimedia Commons, < http://en.wikipedia.org/wiki/Salt#mediaviewer/ File:DeadSeaIsrael5.jpg>

Page 30 Photo Purchased from BigStockPhoto.net

Page 31 Photo By Pixabay user Byrev, <http://pixabay.com/en/drinking-sun-water-woman-young-87155/>

Page 35 Photo Courtesy of FreeDigitalPhotos.net

Page 40 Photo Courtesy of FreeDigitalPhotos.net

Page 42 Photo Courtesy of FreeDigitalPhotos.net

Page 46 Photo Courtesy of FreeDigitalPhotos.net

Page 48 Photo Courtesy of FreeDigitalPhotos.net

Page 55 Photo Courtesy of FreeDigitalPhotos.net

Page 56 Photo Purchased from BigStockPhoto.net

Page 57 Photo Purchased from BigStockPhoto.net

Page 58 Photo Purchased from BigStockPhoto.net

Page 69 Photo Purchased from BigStockPhoto.net

Page 76 Photo Purchased from BigStockPhoto.net

Page 86 Photo Purchased from BigStockPhoto.net

Page 102 Photo Courtesy of FreeDigitalPhotos.net

Page 108 Photo Purchased from BigStockPhoto.net

Page 110 Photo Courtesy of FreeDigitalPhotos.net

Page 112 Photo Courtesy GemRockAuctions.com,
<http://www.gemrockauctions.com/learn/gemstone-
articles/himalayan-salt-lamp-benefits>

Index

S

T

CPSIA information can be obtained at www.ICGtesting.com
Printed in the USA
BVOW11s0526040216

435314BV00012B/63/P